'Mudras for Curing Cancer'

21 Simple Hand Gestures for Preventing & Curing Cancer

Advait

© 2014, Advait, All Rights Reserved

Disclaimer and FTC Notice

Mudras for Curing Cancer: 21 Simple Hand Gestures for Preventing & Curing Cancer
Copyright © 2014, Advait. All Rights Reserved.

ISBN-13: 978-1512247398

ISBN-10: 1512247391

All rights reserved. This book should not be reproduced in any form without permission in writing from the author. Reviewers may quote brief passages in reviews.

No part of this publication may be reproduced or transmitted in any form or by any means, mechanical or electronic, including photocopying or recording, or by any information storage and retrieval system, or transmitted by email without permission in writing from the publisher.

While all attempts have been made to verify the information provided in this publication, neither the author nor the publisher assumes any responsibility for errors, omissions, or contrary interpretations of the subject matter herein.

The author of this book does not dispense medical advice or prescribe the use of any technique as a form of treatment for physical, emotional, or medical problems without the advice of a physician, either directly or indirectly.

The intent of the author is only to offer information of a general nature to help you in your quest for emotional, spiritual and physical well being. In the event you use any of the information in this book for yourself, which is your constitutional right, the author and the publisher assume no responsibility for your actions.

Under no circumstances will any legal responsibility or blame be held against the publisher for any reparation, damages, or monetary loss due to the information herein, either directly or indirectly. The information herein is offered for informational purposes solely, and is universal as so. The presentation of the information is without contract or any type of guarantee assurance.

Adherence to all applicable laws and regulations, including international, federal, state, and local governing professional licensing, business practices, advertising, and all other aspects of doing business in the US, Canada, or any other jurisdiction is the sole responsibility of the purchaser or reader.

Neither the author nor the publisher assumes any responsibility or liability whatsoever on the behalf of the purchaser or reader of these materials.

Any perceived slight of any individual or organization is purely unintentional.

Advait

Contents

What are Mudras? 6

Attention!! 10

How to Use These Mudras? 11

Mudra #1 13

Mudra #2 15

Mudra #3 17

Mudra #4 19

Mudra #5 22

Mudra #6 24

Mudra #7 26

Mudra #8 28

Mudra #9 30

Mudra #10 32

Mudra #11 34

Mudra #12 36

Mudra #13 38

Mudra #14 40

Mudra #15 42

Mudra #16 44

Mudra #17 46

Mudra #18 50

Mudra #19 52

Mudras for Curing Cancer

Mudra #20 54
Mudra #21 57
Thank You 59
Other Books by Advait 60

Advait

What are Mudras?

According to the Vedic culture of ancient India, our entire world is made of 'the five elements' called as *The Panch-Maha-Bhuta's*. The five elements being **Earth**, **Water**, **Fire**, **Wind** and **Space/Vacuum**. They are also called the earth element, water element, fire element, wind element and space element.

These five elements constitute the human body – the nutrients from the soil (earth) are absorbed by the plants which we consume (thus we survive on the earth element), the blood flowing through own veins represents the water element, the body heat represents the fire element, the oxygen we inhale and the carbon dioxide we exhale represents the wind element and the sinuses we have in our nose and skull represent the space element.

As long as these five elements in our body are balanced and maintain appropriate levels we remain healthy. An imbalance of these elements in the human body leads to a deteriorated health and diseases.

Now understand this, the command and control center of all these five elements lies in our fingers. So literally, our health lies at our fingertips.

The Mudra healing method that I am going to teach you depends on our fingers.

To understand this, we should first know the finger-element relationship:

Thumb – Fire element.

Index finger – Wind element.

Middle finger – Space/Vacuum element.

Third finger – Earth element.

Small finger – Water element.

Advait

This image will give you a better understanding of the concept:

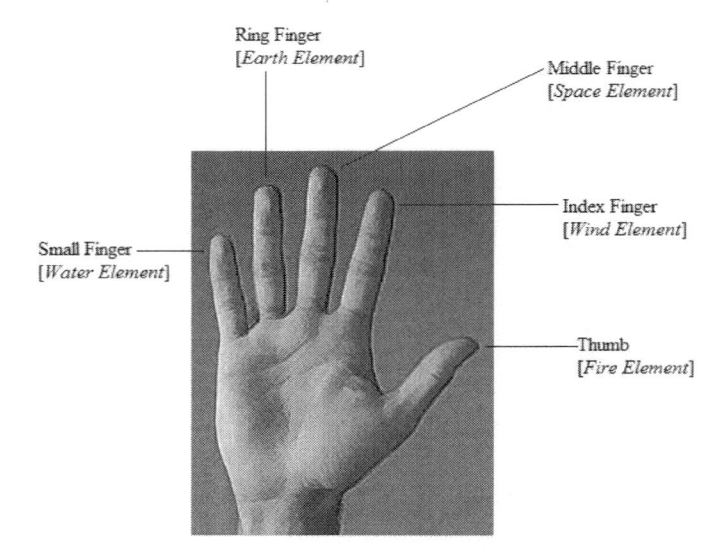

Ring Finger
[*Earth Element*]

Middle Finger
[*Space Element*]

Index Finger
[*Wind Element*]

Small Finger
[*Water Element*]

Thumb
[*Fire Element*]

When the fingers are brought together in a specific pattern and are touched to each other, or slightly pressed against each other, the formation is called as a *'Mudra'*.

When the five fingers are touched and pressed in a peculiar way to form a Mudra, it affects the levels of the five elements in our body, thus balancing those elements and inducing good health.

P.S. The Mudra Healing Methods aren't just theory or wordplay; these are healing methods from the ancient Indian Vedic culture, proven and tested over ages.

Attention!!

Read this before you read any further

For the better understanding of the reader, detail images have been provided for every mudra along with the method to perform it.

Most of the Mudras given in this book are to be performed using both your hands, but the Mudras whose images show only one hand performing the Mudra, are to be performed simultaneously on both your hands for the Mudras to have the maximum effect.

Mudras for Curing Cancer

How to Use These Mudras?

The Mudras Mentioned in this book for preventing & curing Cancer can be classified into three categories, viz.

- a) Mudras for Physical Healing,(Primary Mudras)
- b) Mudras for Emotional Healing and, (Secondary Mudras)
- c) Mudras for Spiritual Healing (Secondary Mudras).

The Mudras for physical healing are the first 14 Mudras (Mudra #1 through Mudra #14), the Mudras for emotional healing and emotional comfort are the next 5 Mudras (Mudra #15 through Mudra #19) and the Final 2 Mudras (Mudra #20 & #21) are used for spiritual healing.

The Mudras for physical healing are to be used regularly and extensively while the Mudras for emotional and spiritual healing are to be used for garnering the required emotional support and stability during the course of Healing and these secondary Mudras increase the healing effects of the Primary Mudras manifolds.

Make sure that you perform all the Primary Mudras regularly and extensively, while performing a few Secondary Mudras regularly which will enhance the effect of the Primary Mudras.

Also, understand that <u>it is NOT a hard and fast rule that you should perform all these 21 Mudras back to back in one session</u>.

Take your time, and perform these Mudras at your own pace and convenience.

The beauty of Mudra Health and Healing Techniques is that Mudras can be performed at any time and place: while stuck in traffic, at the office, watching TV, or whenever you have to twiddle your thumbs waiting for something or someone.

Mudra #1

Mahakraantmudra / Mudra of Supreme Power

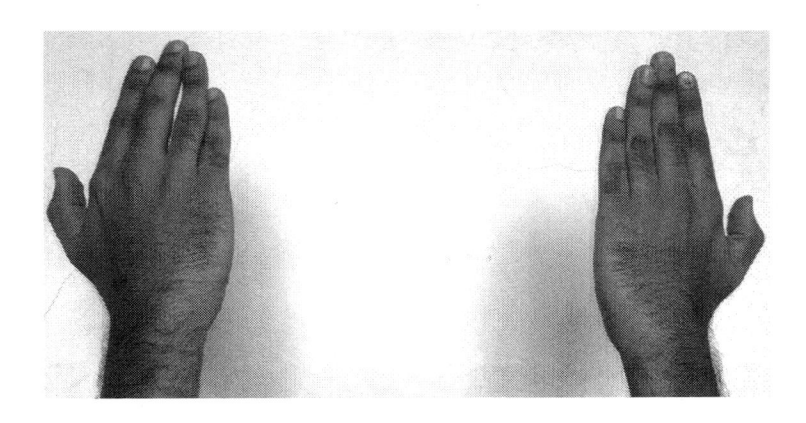

Method:

This Mudra is to be performed in a seated position, preferably facing east.

Be seated comfortably in an upright posture and concentrate on your breathing to relax.

Raise your hands in front of your face with the palms facing you.

Keep both the hands parallel to each other, shoulder width apart.

Feel your hands getting warm, and visualize the light of the rising sun falling on your hands and illuminating them.

Then imagine this stream of light, entering into your face and flowing into your entire body from there.

Duration:

This Mudra should be performed for at least 5 minutes and can be performed for 15 minutes at a stretch.

This Mudra should be performed twice a day, once in the morning and once in the evening for best results.

Mudra #2

Mudgaramudra / Mudra of Club

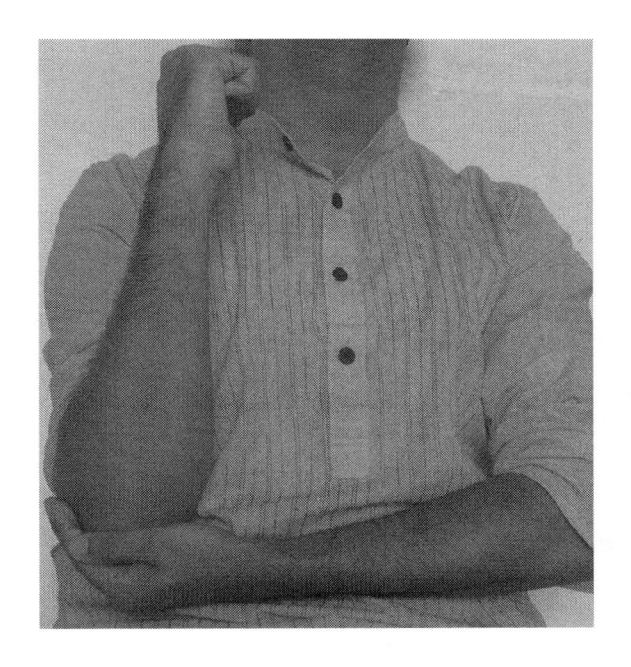

Method:

This Mudra is to be performed in a seated position.

Be seated comfortably in an upright posture and concentrate on your breathing to relax.

Advait

Form a fist with your right hand and rest the right elbow on the left palm.

(Refer the image)

Relax the shoulders and breathe comfortably.

Duration:

This Mudra should be performed for at least 5 minutes and can be performed for 30 minutes at a stretch.

This Mudra should be performed twice a day, once in the morning and once in the evening for best results.

Mudras for Curing Cancer

Mudra #3

Granthitamudra / Mudra of Glands

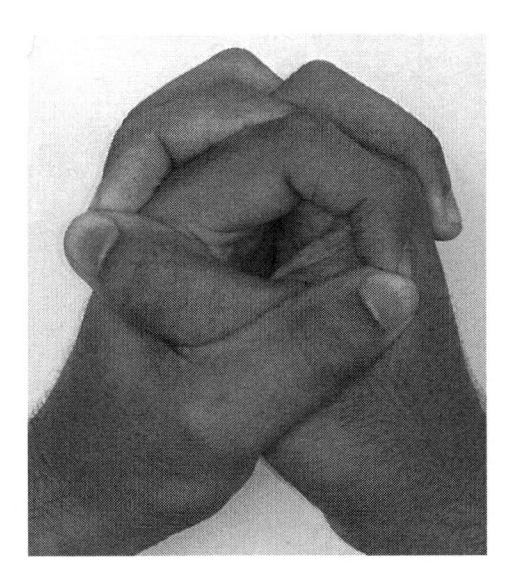

Method:

This Mudra is to be performed in a seated position.

Be seated comfortably in an upright posture and concentrate on your breathing to relax.

Clasp both your hands together as shown in the image.

Note that the left index figure is on top of the right index finger.

Now, join the tips of the Index finger and Thumb of the respective hands together.

Hold this Mudra in front of your Throat.

Duration:

This Mudra should be performed for at least 5 minutes and can be performed for 40 minutes at a stretch.

This Mudra should be performed twice a day, once in the morning and once in the evening for best results.

Mudra #4

Tritiiya Kurmamudra / Mudra of Tortoise III

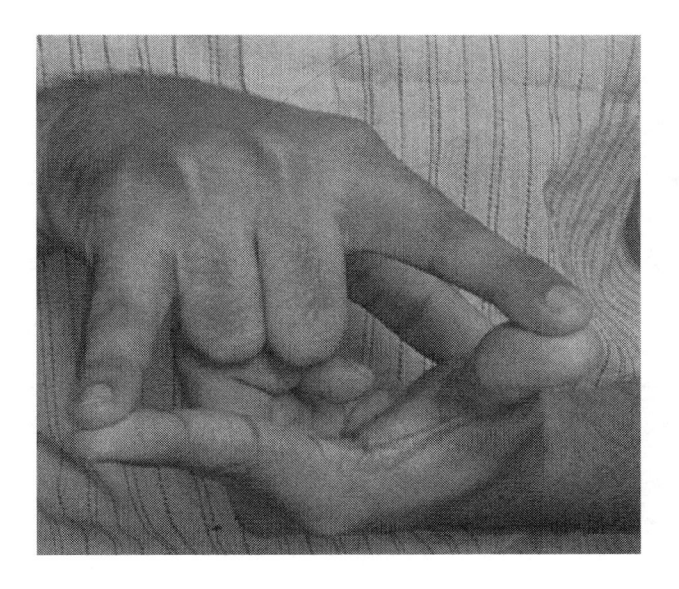

Method:

This Mudra is to be performed in a seated position.

Be seated comfortably in an upright posture and concentrate on your breathing to relax.

Advait

Raise your palms to chest height, with the left palm facing upwards while the right palm is facing downwards.

Curl down the Middle, Ring and Little fingers of the left hand to form a partial fist, while keeping the Index finger and Thumb extended.

Curl down the Middle and ring fingers of the right hand to form a partial fist, while keeping the Index finger, Little finger and the Thumb extended.

Now, keep the right palm over the left palm.

Then,

Touch the tip of the right Index finger to the tip of the left thumb.

Touch the tip of the right Little finger to the tip of the left Index finger.

Touch the tip of the right Thumb to the base of the left Thumb near the wrist.

After forming this Mudra, hold this Mudra in front of your Solar Plexus (just below your sternum)

Duration:

Mudras for Curing Cancer

This Mudra should be performed for at least 5 minutes and can be performed for 40 minutes at a stretch.

This Mudra should be performed twice a day, once in the morning and once in the evening for best results.

Mudra #5

Shanmukhamudra / Mudra of Six Faces

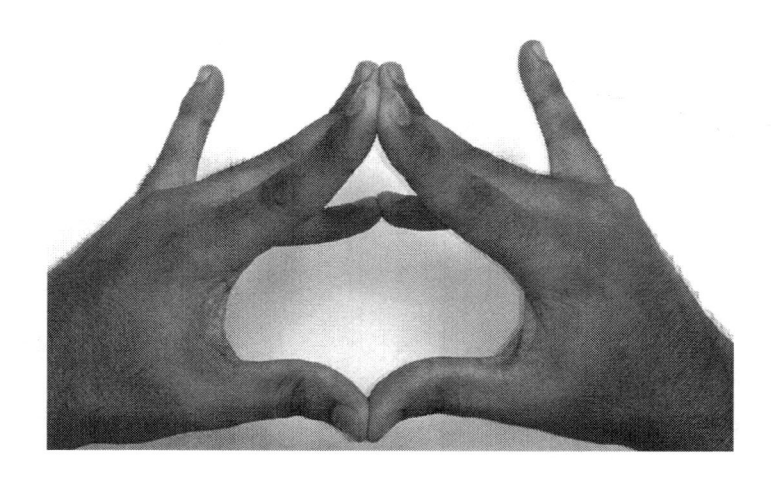

Method:

This Mudra is to be performed in a seated position.

Be seated comfortably in an upright posture and concentrate on your breathing to relax.

Hold your palms in front of your chest facing each other.

Mudras for Curing Cancer

Now extend all the fingers on both the hands outwards.

Then, touch tips of all fingers of one hand to the tips of the respective fingers of the other hand, except the ring fingers.

Keep both the Ring fingers extended outwards.

(Refer the image)

Once the Mudra is formed lower the Mudra hold it in front of your abdomen.

Duration:

This Mudra should be performed for at least 5 minutes and can be performed for 40 minutes at a stretch.

This Mudra should be performed twice a day, once in the morning and once in the evening for best results.

Mudra #6

Vistaaramudra / Mudra of Expansion

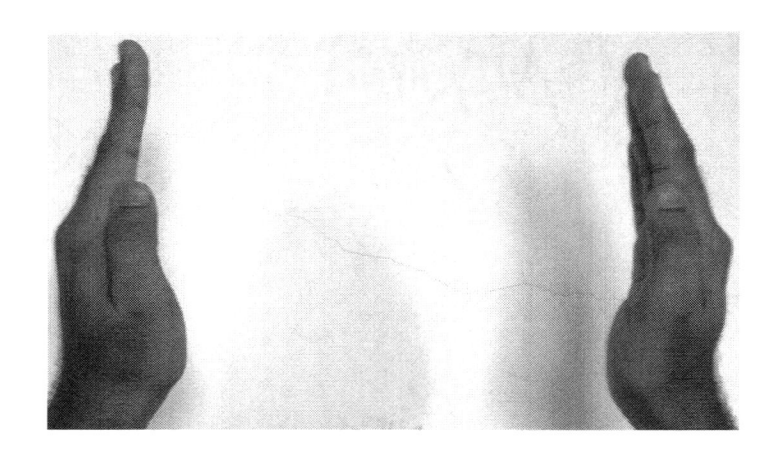

Method:

This Mudra is to be performed in a seated position.

Be seated comfortably in an upright posture and concentrate on your breathing to relax.

Bring both your hands in front of your belly with your palms facing each other.

Mudras for Curing Cancer

Keep the palms around 10 inches apart from each other.

Close your eyes and then as you inhale and as your belly inflates increase the distance between your palms by an inch, then when you exhale and as your belly deflates bring the palms closer by an inch.

Duration:

This Mudra should be performed for at least 5 minutes and can be performed for 20 minutes at a stretch.

This Mudra should be performed twice a day, once in the morning and once in the evening for best results.

Mudra #7

Abhayhridaymudra / Mudra of Assured Heart

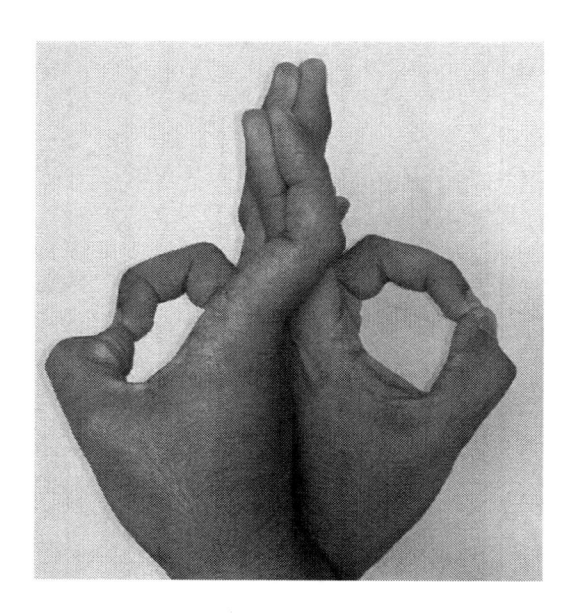

Method:

This Mudra is to be performed in a seated position.

Be seated comfortably in an upright posture and concentrate on your breathing to relax.

Mudras for Curing Cancer

Join your palms together as in the Indian form of salutation 'Namaste'.

Now cross the palms at your wrist, with the back of the palms facing each other and the wrist of the right hand closer to the body.

Interlock the Index, Middle and Little fingers at the tips. (Refer the image)

Join the tips of the Ring fingers and the Thumbs as shown in the image.

Duration:

This Mudra should be performed for at least 5 minutes and can be performed for 45 minutes at a stretch.

This Mudra should be performed twice a day, once in the morning and once in the evening for best results.

Advait

Mudra #8

Mritsanjeevanimudra (Apaanvayumudra) / Mudra of Resurrection

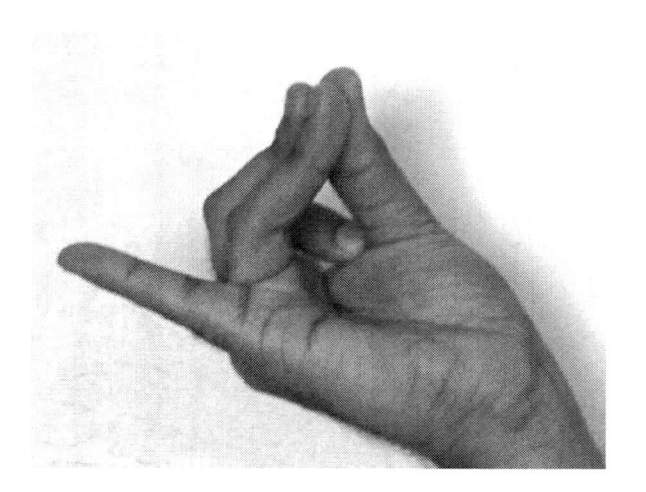

Method:

This Mudra is to be performed in a seated position.

Be seated comfortably in an upright posture and concentrate on your breathing to relax.

Touch the base of your Thumb with the tip of the Index finger and press slightly.

Then, touch the tips of the Index finger, Middle finger and Thumb together.

Keep the Little finger extended outwards.

Perform the Mudra's on both your hands and place them on your thighs.

Duration:

This Mudra should be performed for at least 5 minutes and can be performed for 40 minutes at a stretch.

This Mudra should be performed twice a day, once in the morning and once in the evening for best results.

Mudra #9

Sinhkraantamudra / Mudra of Lion's Paw

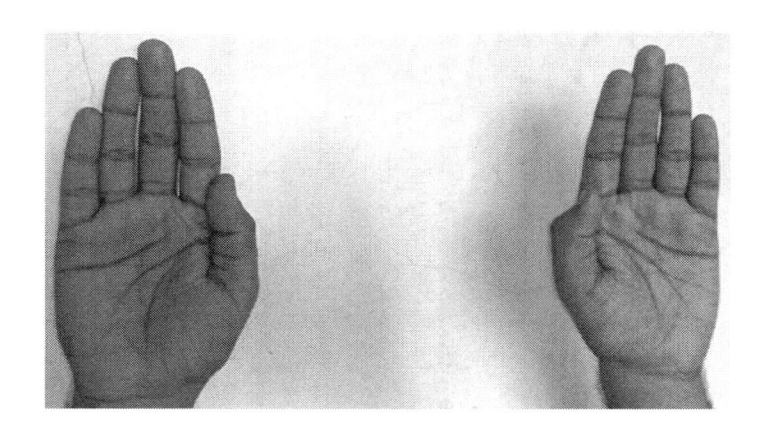

Method:

This Mudra is to be performed in a seated position.

Be seated comfortably in an upright posture and concentrate on your breathing to relax.

Lift your palms at shoulder height with the palms facing away from you.

Mudras for Curing Cancer

Extend all the fingers upwards, and touching each other at the sides.

(Refer the image)

Hold this Mudra at the shoulder level.

Duration:

This Mudra should be performed for at least 5 minutes and can be performed for 30 minutes at a stretch.

This Mudra should be performed twice a day, once in the morning and once in the evening for best results.

Mudra #10

Vititamudra / Mudra of Blooming

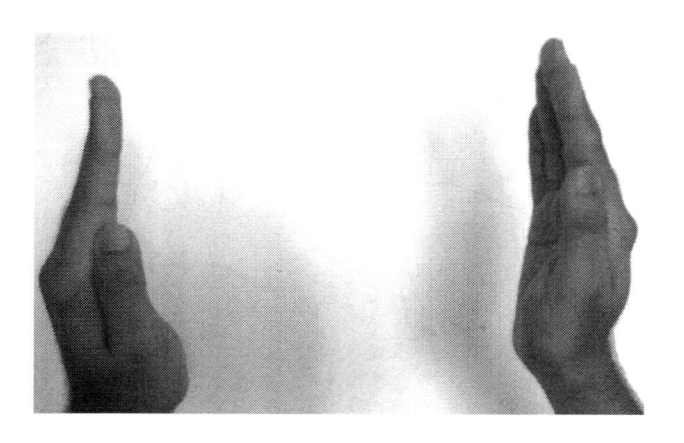

Method:

This Mudra is a variation of the *'Vistaaramudra'*.

This Mudra is to be performed in a seated position.

Be seated comfortably in an upright posture and concentrate on your breathing to relax.

Bring both your hands in front of your belly with your palms facing each other.

Keep the palms around **3 inches apart** from each other.

Close your eyes and then as you inhale and as your belly inflates increase the distance between your palms by an inch, then when you exhale and as your belly deflates bring the palms closer by an inch.

Duration:

This Mudra should be performed for at least 5 minutes and can be performed for 20 minutes at a stretch.

This Mudra should be performed twice a day, once in the morning and once in the evening for best results.

Advait

Mudra #11

Samputamudra / Mudra of Bud

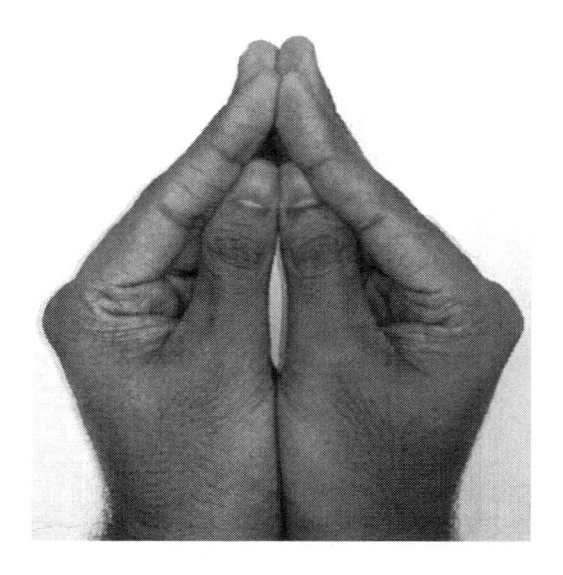

Method:

It's a modified form of the 'Prayer Mudra'.

This Mudra is to be performed in a seated position.

Be seated comfortably in an upright posture and concentrate on your breathing to relax.

Touch the tip of the fingers of your right hand with the tip of the fingers of your left hand as shown in the image.

Make hollow space between both the palms as if you are holding a small bird.

Now, take this formation in front of your eyes, and look through the hollow space and concentrate on your breathing for a couple of minutes, then hold this Mudra in front of your Heart.

Duration:

This Mudra should be performed for at least 5 minutes and can be performed for 30 minutes at a stretch.

This Mudra should be performed twice a day, once in the morning and once in the evening for best results.

Mudra #12

Pallavamudra / Mudra of Leaf Swaying on Wind

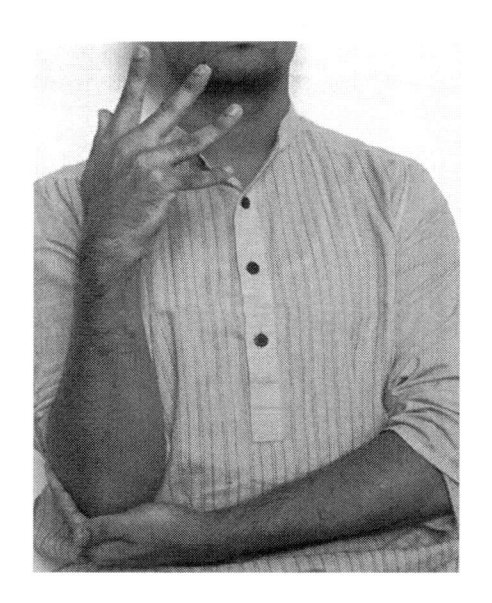

Method:

This Mudra is to be performed in a seated position.

Be seated comfortably in an upright posture and concentrate on your breathing to relax.

Mudras for Curing Cancer

Now, raise your right palm to shoulder height and rest the right elbow on your left palm.

Your right palm should be facing you.

Relax the right palm completely and let the fingers of the right hand move freely as if they are leaves swaying in wind.

Visualize your left palm as the earth (ground) while your right hand as the tree with your fingers of the right hand as the leaves of the tree swaying freely on the wind.

Duration:

This Mudra should be performed for at least 5 minutes and can be performed for 30 minutes at a stretch.

This Mudra should be performed twice a day, once in the morning and once in the evening for best results.

Advait

Mudra #13

Chonmukha Mukhamudra / Mudra of Up and Down Face

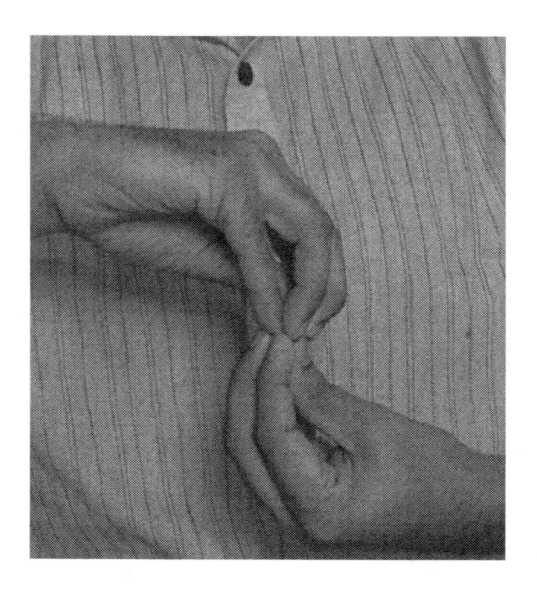

Method:

This Mudra is to be performed in a seated position.

Be seated comfortably in an upright posture and concentrate on your breathing to relax.

Mudras for Curing Cancer

Raise both your hands to chest height with both the palms facing upwards.

Collect the fingers of each hand in such a way that pads of the Thumbs lightly touch the pads of the other four fingers.

Now, with the left palm facing down and the right palm facing up, touch both these Mudras at the fingertips.

After 5-10 minutes reverse the Mudra, i.e. Left palm should face up and the right palm should face down and hold this Position for another 5-10 minutes.

While doing both the variations of this Mudra, touch the tip of your tongue to your upper palate. (This will significantly increase the benefits of this Mudra.)

Duration:

Each variation of this Mudra should be performed for at least 5 minutes and can be performed for 10 minutes at a stretch.

This Mudra should be performed twice a day, once in the morning and once in the evening for best results.

Advait

Mudra #14

Tritiiya Varahamudra / Mudra of Hog III

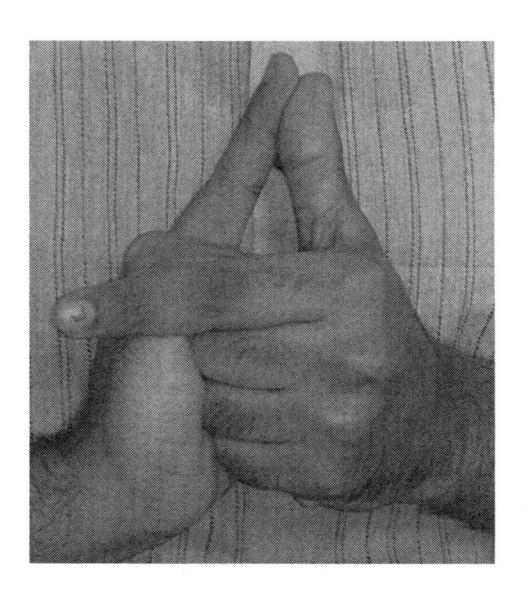

Method:

This Mudra is to be performed in a seated position.

Be seated comfortably in an upright posture and concentrate on your breathing to relax.

Mudras for Curing Cancer

Hold your left hand in front of your chest, palm facing you.

Curl the Middle, Ring and Little finger of the left hand inwards.

The Index finger should be pointing towards right and the Thumb should be extended upwards.

Now, clasp the curled fingers of the left hand with the fingers of the right hand.

Then, touch the tip of the Thumb of your left hand with the tip of the Index finger of your right hand.

Touch the tip of your right Thumb to the base of the left Thumb.

The Left Index finger should be resting outside the right Little finger.

Duration:

This Mudra should be performed for at least 5 minutes and can be performed for 45 minutes at a stretch.

This Mudra should be performed twice a day, once in the morning and once in the evening for best results.

Advait

Mudra #15

Hridaymudra / Mudra of Heart

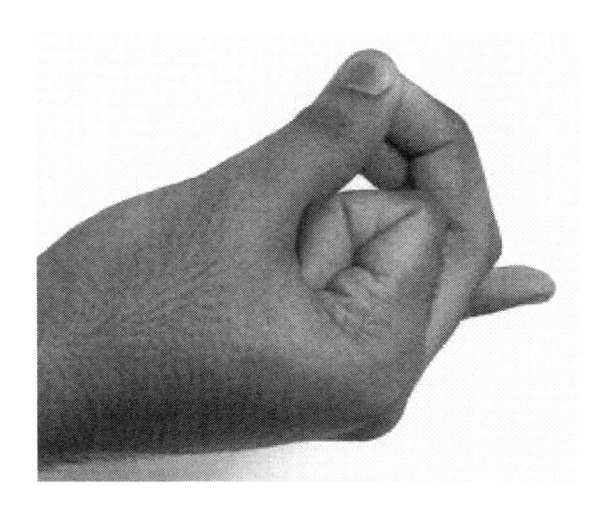

Method:

This Mudra is to be performed in a seated position.

Be seated comfortably in an upright posture and concentrate on your breathing to relax.

Try to touch the base of the Index finger with the tip of the same Index finger.

Mudras for Curing Cancer

Now, roll this bent Index finger forward in such a way that the first knuckle of the Index finger touches the base of the Thumb (Refer the image).

Now join the tips of the Thumb, Middle and Ring fingers together and press slightly.

Keep the Little finger outstretched.

This Mudra is to be performed on both your palms simultaneously and then rest this Mudras on your thighs.

Duration:

This Mudra should be performed for at least 5 minutes and can be performed for 40 minutes at a stretch.

This Mudra should be performed twice a day, once in the morning and once in the evening for best results.

Advait

Mudra #16

Prithvimudra / Mudra of Earth

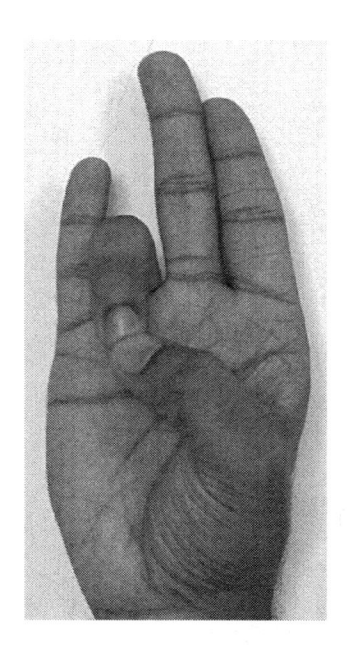

Method:

This Mudra is to be performed in a sitting position.

Be seated comfortably in an upright posture and concentrate on your breathing to relax.

Mudras for Curing Cancer

Place your palms in your lap, facing upwards.

Join the tips of your Ring finger and Thumb together and press slightly.

Keep all the other fingers extended outwards.

Duration:

This Mudra should be performed for at least 5 minutes and can be performed for 45 minutes at a stretch.

This Mudra should be performed twice a day, once in the morning and once in the evening for best results.

Mudra #17

AnaahatChakramudra / Mudra of Un-struck Hymn

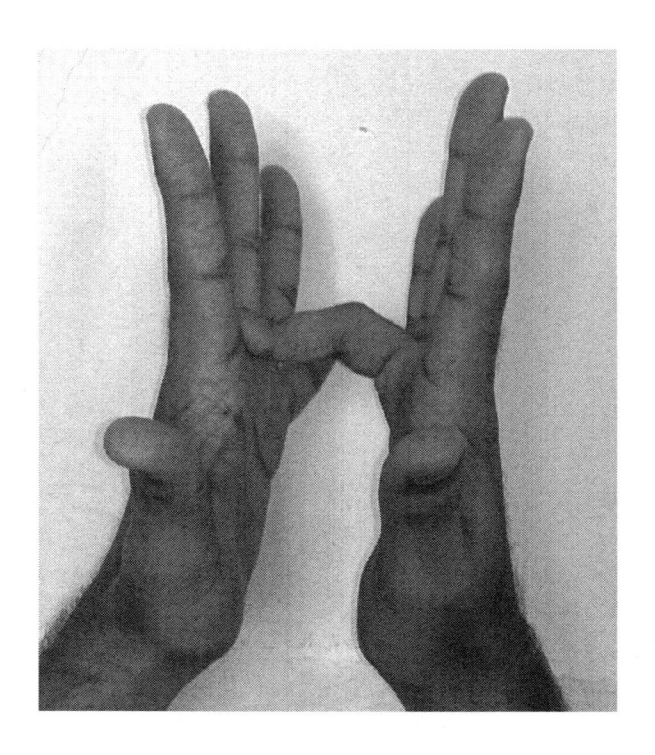

Mudras for Curing Cancer

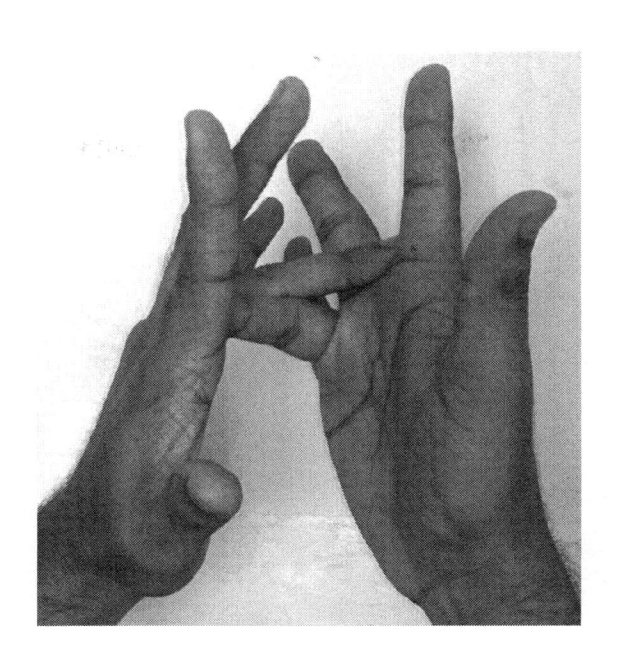

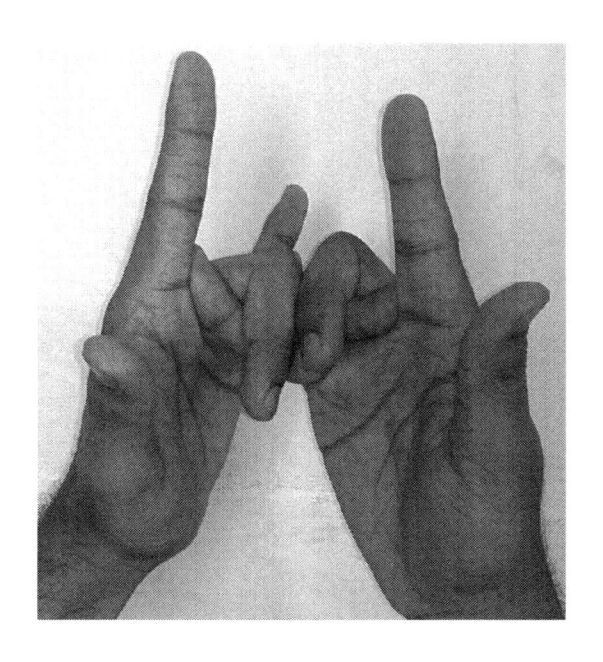

Advait

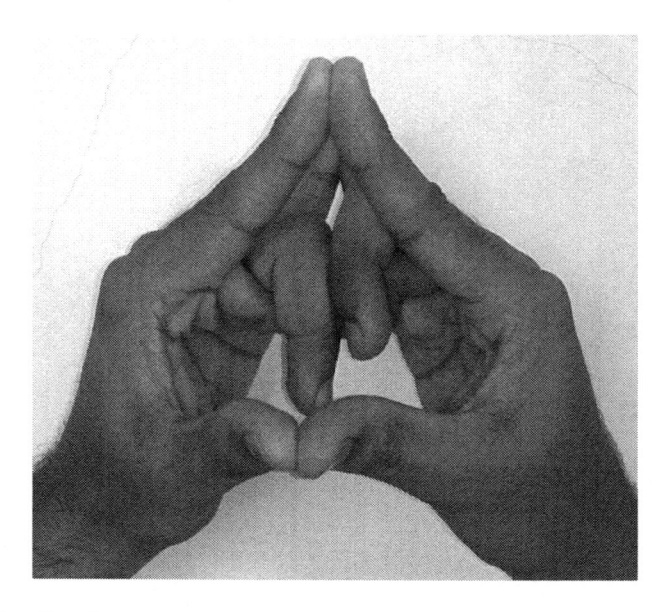

Method:

This Mudra is to be performed in a seated position.

Be seated comfortably in an upright posture and concentrate on your breathing to relax.

Place the right Ring finger on the web between the Index and Middle finger of the left hand.

Place the left Ring finger on the web between the Index and Middle finger of the right hand.

Curl down both the middle fingers to wrap and press down the respective Ring fingers of the opposite hands.

Mudras for Curing Cancer

Now join the tips of both the Index and Little fingers together, outstretch them and press slightly.

Then join the tips of both the Thumbs together, outstretch them and press slightly.

This Mudra is to be held in front of your chest.

Duration:

This Mudra should be performed for at least 5 minutes and can be performed for 40 minutes at a stretch.

This Mudra should be performed twice a day, once in the morning and once in the evening for best results.

Mudra #18

Mushtimudra / Mudra of Fist

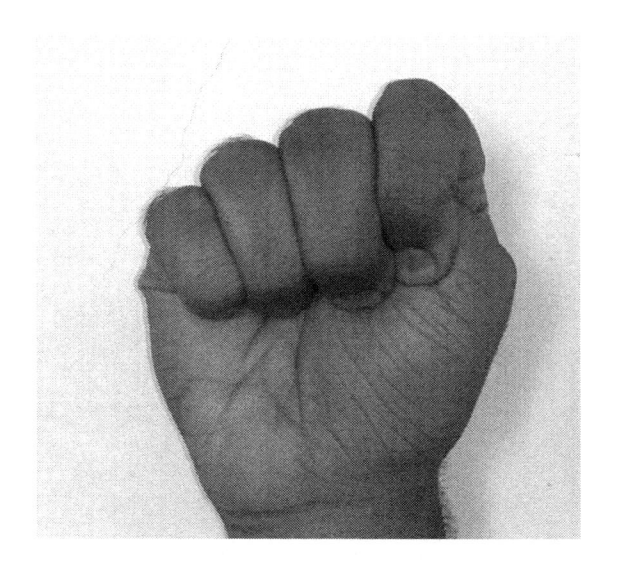

Method:

This Mudra is to be performed in a seated position.

Be seated comfortably in an upright posture and concentrate on your breathing to relax.

Touch the tip of your thumb to the base of the Ring finger and press slightly.

Close all the other fingers over the Thumb to form a fist.

(Refer the image)

Form this Mudra on each hand and rest the fists against the lower belly.

Duration:

This Mudra should be performed for at least 5 minutes and can be performed for 40 minutes at a stretch.

This Mudra should be performed twice a day, once in the morning and once in the evening for best results.

Mudra #19

Shukrimudra / Mudra of Purity

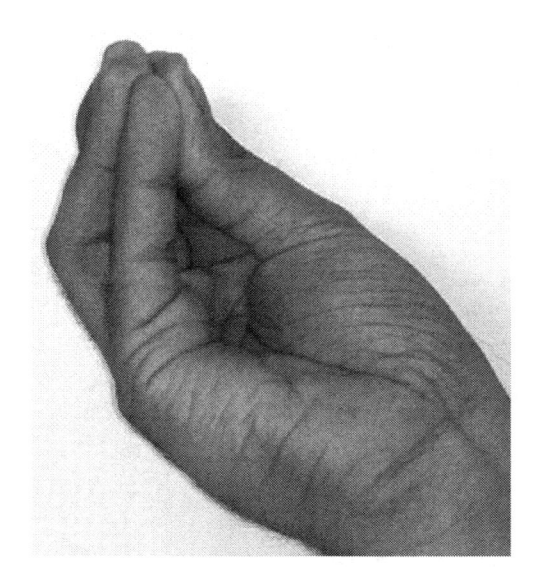

Method:

This Mudra can be performed while being seated, in a standing position or lying in bed.

Concentrate on your breathing to relax and feel comfortable.

Mudras for Curing Cancer

Join the tips of all your fingers together to make this Mudra. (Refer the image)

Your palms should be facing upwards.

For best results perform this Mudra lying down.

Duration:

This Mudra should be performed for at least 5 minutes and can be performed for 30 minutes at a stretch.

This Mudra should be performed twice a day, once in the morning and once in the evening for best results.

Mudra #20

Mandalamudra / Mudra of Orbit

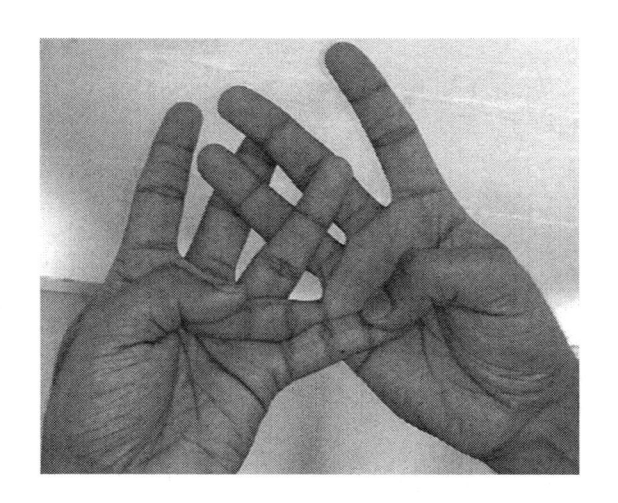

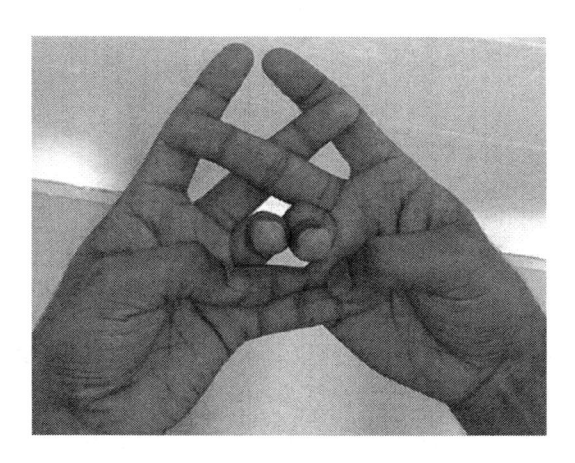

Mudras for Curing Cancer

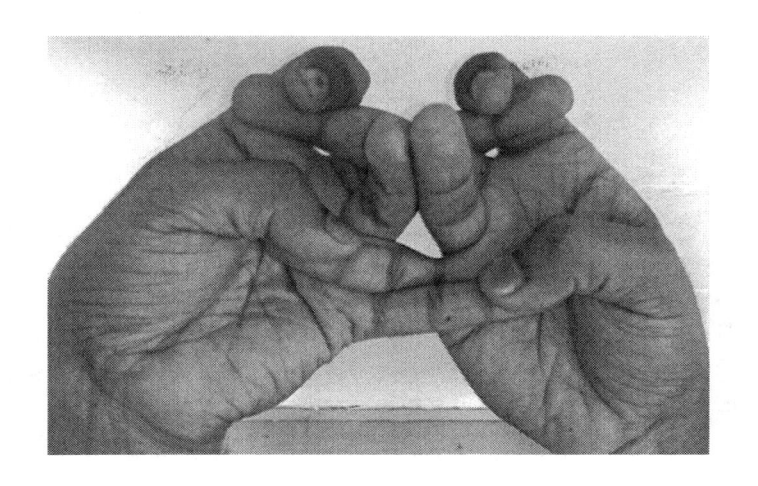

Method:

This Mudra is to be performed in a seated position.

Be seated comfortably in an upright posture and concentrate on your breathing to relax.

Keep your palms at chest height, facing upwards.

Cross both the Little fingers and press them down with opposite Thumbs.

Keep both the Ring fingers extended and outstretched, pointing upwards and touching each other adjacently.

Then cross both the Middle fingers and press them down with opposite Index fingers.

Advait

Hold this Mudra in front of your Sternum.

Duration:

This Mudra should be performed for at least 5 minutes and can be performed for 45 minutes at a stretch.

This Mudra should be performed twice a day, once in the morning and once in the evening for best results.

Mudra #21

DharmaChakramudra / Mudra of Wheel of Dharma

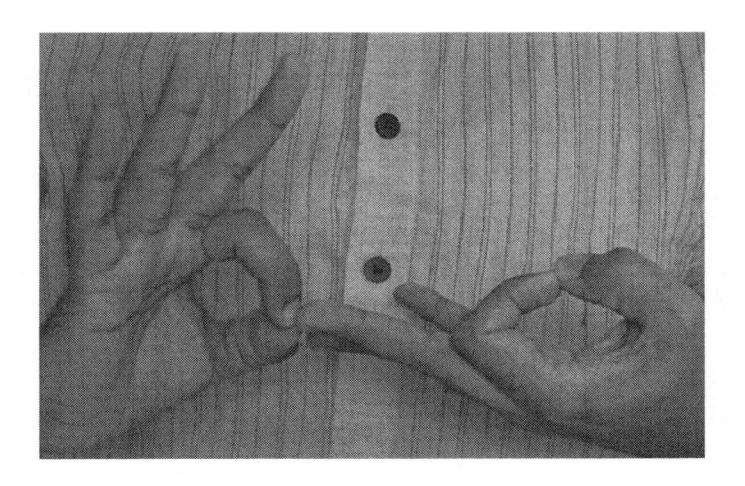

Method:

This Mudra is to be performed in a seated position.

Be seated comfortably in an upright posture and concentrate on your breathing to relax.

Join the tips of Thumb and Index fingers on both the hands.

Advait

With the hands in front of your chest (Heart) touch the touch the tip of the Middle finger of the left hand to the tips of the Thumb and Index finger of the right hand.

Your right palm should face forward while your left palm should face your body.

Duration:

This Mudra should be performed for at least 5 minutes and can be performed for 45 minutes at a stretch.

This Mudra should be performed twice a day, once in the morning and once in the evening for best results.

Thank You

Thank you so much for reading my book. I hope you really liked it.

As you probably know, many people look at the reviews on Amazon before they decide to purchase a book.

If you liked the book, please take a minute to leave a review with your feedback.

60 seconds is all I'm asking for, and it would mean a lot to me.

Thank You so much.

All the best,

Advait

Other Books by Advait

Mudras for Awakening Chakras: 19 Simple Hand Gestures for Awakening & Balancing Your Chakras

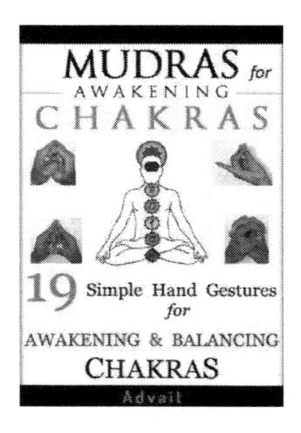

http://www.amazon.com/dp/B00P82COAY

[#1 Bestseller in 'Yoga']

[#1 Bestseller in 'Chakras']

Mudras for Curing Cancer

Mudras for Weight Loss: 21 Simple Hand Gestures for Effortless Weight Loss

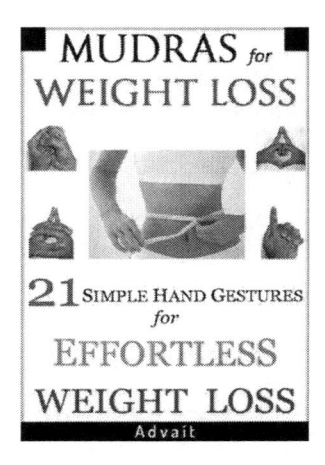

http://www.amazon.com/dp/B00P3ZPSEK

Advait

Mudras for Spiritual Healing: 21 Simple Hand Gestures for Ultimate Spiritual Healing & Awakening

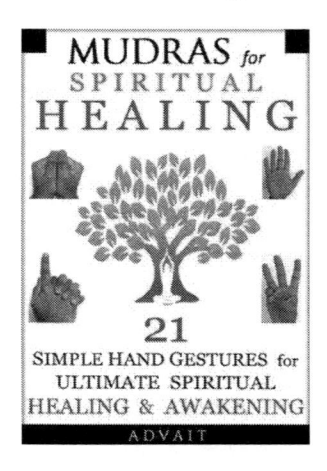

http://www.amazon.com/dp/B00PFYZLQO

Mudras for Curing Cancer

Mudras for Sex: 25 Simple Hand Gestures for Extreme Erotic Pleasure & Sexual Vitality

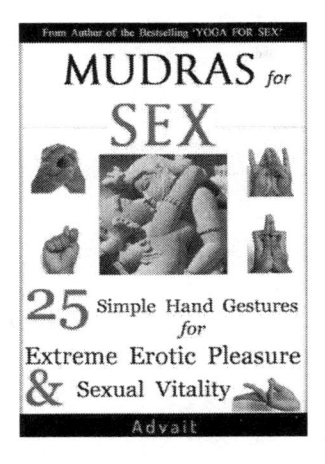

http://www.amazon.com/dp/B00OJR1DRY

Mudras: 25 Ultimate Techniques for Self Healing

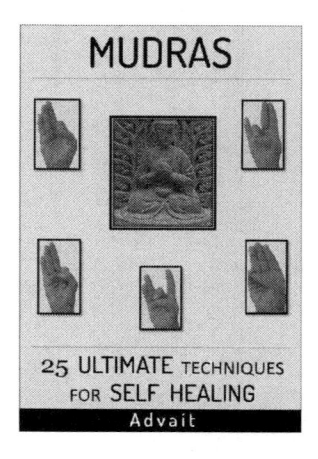

http://www.amazon.com/dp/B00MMPB5CI

Mudras for Curing Cancer

Mudras of Anxiety: 25 Simple Hand Gestures for Curing Anxiety

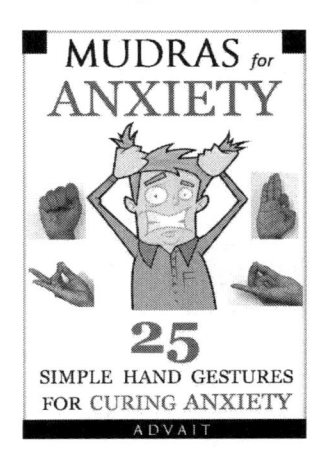

http://www.amazon.com/dp/B00PF011IU

Mudras for a Strong Heart: 21 Simple Hand Gestures for Preventing, Curing & Reversing Heart Disease

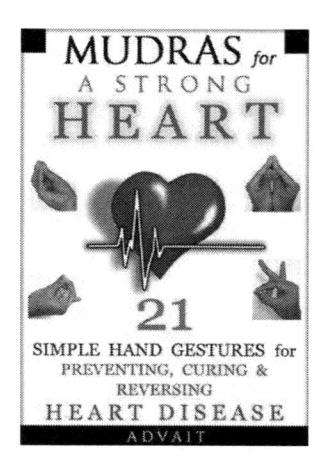

http://www.amazon.com/dp/B00PFRLGTM

Mudras for Curing Cancer

Mudras for Stress Management: 21 Simple Hand Gestures for a Stress Free Life

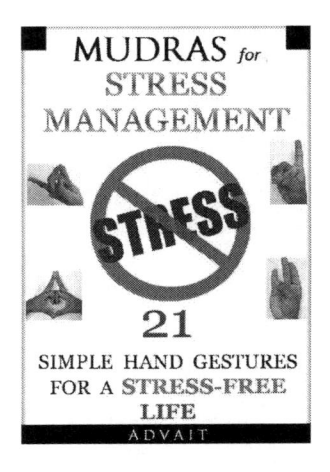

http://amazon.com/dp/B00PFTJ6OC

Mudras for Memory Improvement: 25 Simple Hand Gestures for Ultimate Memory Improvement

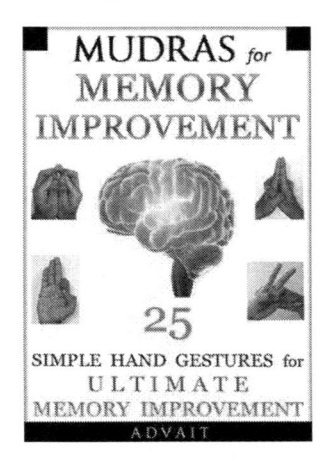

http://www.amazon.com/dp/B00PFSP8TK

Mudras for Curing Cancer

Made in the USA
Middletown, DE
07 May 2017